Lynda AOUDIA

All you need to know about breast calcifications

Lynda AOUDIA

All you need to know about breast calcifications

ScienciaScripts

Imprint

Cover image: www.ingimage.com

This book is a translation from the original published under ISBN 978-620-6-71267-1.

Publisher:
Sciencia Scripts
is a trademark of
Dodo Books Indian Ocean Ltd. and OmniScriptum S.R.L publishing group

120 High Road, East Finchley, London, N2 9ED, United Kingdom
Str. Armeneasca 28/1, office 1, Chisinau MD-2012, Republic of Moldova, Europe
Printed at: see last page
ISBN: 978-620-7-63273-2

EVERYTHING YOU NEED TO KNOW ABOUT BREAST CALCIFICATIONS

LYNDA AOUDIA

FOREWORD

The incidence of breast microcalcifications has increased by around 15-20% since mass screening for breast cancer was introduced. But it has also increased thanks to technological advances in digital mammography, which have made it easier to detect these calcifications. This is a very sensitive sign, but unfortunately its specificity remains low, at less than 20%, and most microcalcifications are benign. However, they represent the most frequent mode of revelation of subclinical cancers. Their discovery poses diagnostic problems, with a constant risk of missing an early-stage cancer, but also of increasing the number of unnecessary surgeries for benign lesions. Microcalcifications require a precise radiological study to determine whether they are benign or malignant.

The aim of this book is to provide a precise description of the morphological mammographic characteristics of calcifications, as well as a study of their distribution in the breast, in order to classify them according to the ACR's BI-RADS classification, which will subsequently determine the most appropriate course of action.

Professor Lynda AOUDIA

TABLE OF CONTENTS

FOREWORD 2

INTRODUCTION 4

MAMMARY ANATOMY AND HISTOLOGY 5

PATHOPHYSIOLOGY 7

PHYSICOCHEMICAL REMINDER 11

MAMMOGRAPHY 12

BI-RADS CALCIFICATION OF THE ACR 17

BI-RADS GLOSSARY 18

ACR BI-RADS MAMMOGRAPHY CLASSIFICATION 34

MAMMARY CALCIFICATIONS AND PATHOLOGIES 35

REFERENCES 55

INTRODUCTION

In breast pathology, there are two types of calcification: microcalcifications and macrocalcifications. By definition, breast microcalcifications correspond to calcium-toned images < 1 mm in size. Those larger than 1 mm are known as macrocalcifications. The size of these calcifications is classically a first element of diagnostic orientation, macrocalcifications being usually benign, even if this is not always verified. Some macrocalcifications, such as linear branch calcifications exceeding one millimetre in size, correspond to a malignant aetiology such as non-specific carcinoma, formerly known as intracanal carcinoma. Microcalcifications represent benign lesions in around 70% of cases, while the remaining 30% are either borderline lesions with a high risk of malignant transformation, such as atypical ductal or lobular hyperplasia, or malignant lesions.

MAMMARY ANATOMY AND HISTOLOGY

1.Breast anatomy

The breast is a globular organ occupying the anterior-superior part of the thorax. It lies on top of the pectoralis muscle, which holds it in place [1]. It is mainly made up of a mammary gland, supporting connective tissue and adipose tissue, all covered by the skin. The top of the breast is represented by the nipple surrounded by the areola (fig. 1). It is made up of around fifteen main milk ducts, each delimiting a lobe. The milk ducts open into the nipple at the level of the milk pores after dilating slightly, forming a lactiferous sinus. Thin fibrous septa separate the lobes, extending into the dermis at the anterior surface of the gland to form Cooper's ligaments, which form Duret's ridges (fig. 1).

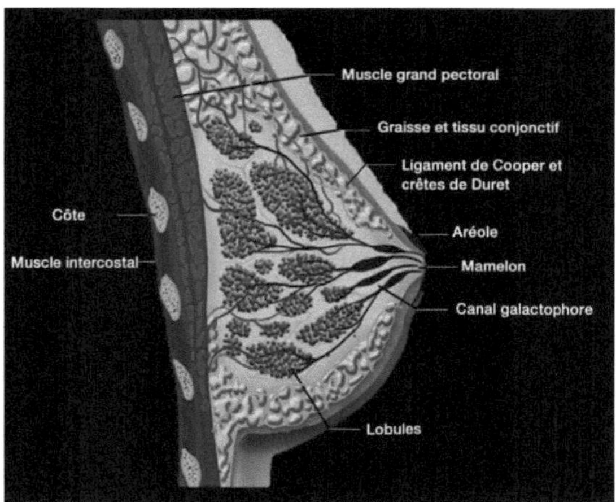

Fig. 1 Anatomical structure of the breast.

2.Galactophoric tree

The breast is made up of around fifteen main milk ducts, ending in a nipple pore. These main ducts, after a dilatation known as the lactiferous sinus, branch off into secondary ducts of medium and small calibre up to the Ductulo-Lobular Terminal Unit (DLTU). This UDTL is made up of a terminal extra- and intra-lobular galactophore and a lobule made up ofaround ten alveoli called acini. The UDTL is embedded in a loose connective tissue known as pallaeal tissue. All of this tissue is surrounded by adipose tissue (fig. 2).

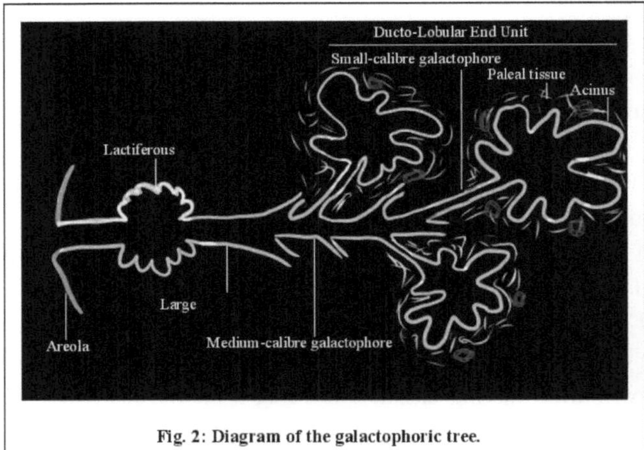

Fig. 2: Diagram of the galactophoric tree.

3.Histological reminder

The whole of the galactophoric tree is made up of a double layer of cells resting on a basement membrane in direct contact with the blood vessels (fig. 3):

- an inner layer made up of cylindrical epithelial cells responsible for the milk secretory function.
- an outer layer made up of myoepithelial cells responsible for contraction.

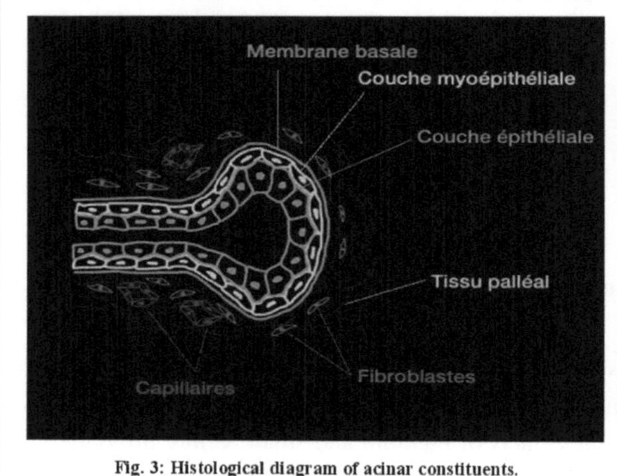

Fig. 3: Histological diagram of acinar constituents.

PATHOPHYSIOLOGY

Intramammary microcalcifications are caused by two phenomena:

- **The secretion of calcium salts by the cylindrical galactophoric epithelium:** The cells lining the galactophores and lobules have a secretory activity (calcium milk), calcifications are due to the accumulation and stagnation of these physiological secretions either by a mechanical effect favouring stasis, such as tumour compression of the galactophore or deformation of the UDTL secondary to fibrocystic dystrophy, or by ultra-structural modification of the galactophoric epithelium, for example in apocrine metaplasia where the production capacity of the cells is increased and their resorption capacity is decreased.
- **Cellular necrosis of altered cells :**

Calcifications arise from calcareous deposits formed in areas of necrosis, most often tumour necrosis.

1.Microcalcification development sector

On the basis of anatomical and histological data, three areas can be identified where microcalcifications will develop:

1.1.Connective tissue

Microcalcifications are due to alterations in the collagen fibres that generally accompany tumourous or non-tumourous disorders of the galactophoric tree, such as the inflammatory fibrosis of benign or scarring mastopathies and the reactive stroma of cancer.

1.2.Galactophoric epithelium

Microcalcifications are then due to the anarchic proliferation of cells, generating metabolic imbalances responsible for cell necrosis. They are found in benign proliferative diseases of the epithelium such as ductal hyperplasia, with or without atypia, and in malignant proliferative diseases.

1.3.Galactophoric ducts

Microcalcifications are linked to the stagnation of secretions leading to calcium precipitation. These are found in fibrocystic dysplasia, especially as the galactophoric epithelium is usually in apocrine metaplasia, which favours secretion but reduces resorption, and also in malignant tumour duct compression.

2.Shape and distribution of microcalcifications

The shape and distribution of microcalcifications are linked to the place where they develop, the mould principle. The calcification mould may correspond to (fig. 4):

- or to a normal structure such as a vessel or sebaceous gland;
- or to the galactophoric tree, at the ductal or lobular level;
- or to a structure neoformed by a pathological process, such as cytosteatonecrosis or a foreign body;
- or by the stroma of a malignant or benign tumour;

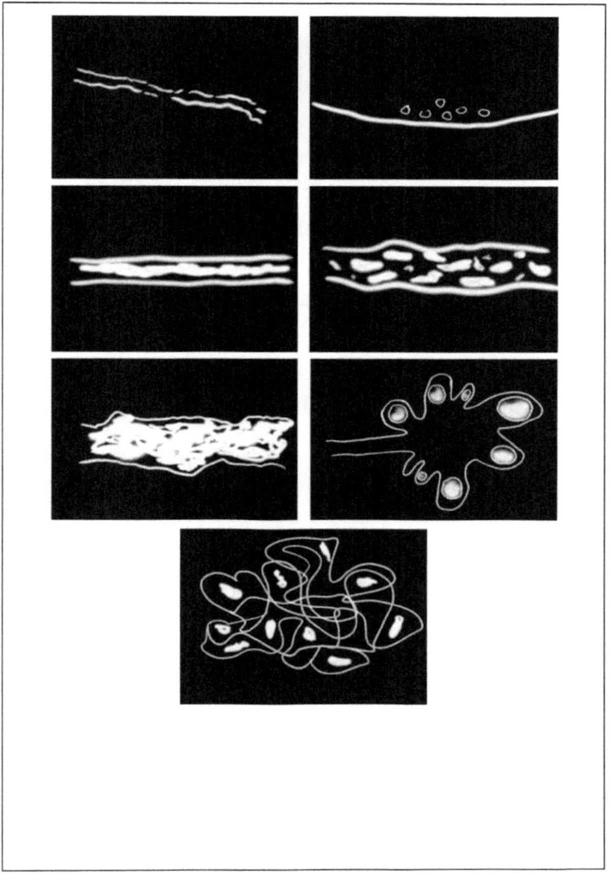

Fig. 4: Diagram showing the shape and distribution of microcalcifications.
(a) Vascular. (b) Sebaceous glands. Ductal calcifications (c) Secretory ectasia. (d) Cribiform carcinoma. (e) Comedocarcinoma. (f) Lobular: fibrocystic dystrophy. (j) Stromal and neoformed structure: cytosteatonecrosis.

There are two types of calcification in the galactophoric tree, depending on where they originate:

- ductal calcifications: these are calcifications which mould the galactophoric duct. They may be linear, branched or ramified. They are distributed linearly or segmentally, sometimes forming a true galactogram. Diagnosis of these calcifications is generally easy and corresponds to two entities, either a secretory ductal ectasia or a ductal carcinoma;

- Lobular calcifications: these are calcifications arising in the lobule. They take on a variety of shapes, most often rounded or dusty, depending on the shape of the lobule and often subject to deformities either related to cystic fibrosis dystrophy or related to a malignant lesion. They are distributed in single or multiple rounded clusters that form the shape of the UDTL. Most often these calcifications are related to a benign pathology, fibrocystic dystrophy, but they can also be related to a malignant pathology by direct proliferation of cancer cells inside the lobule or, on the contrary, by stagnation of calcium secretions due to tumour obstruction of the lobule's drainage pathways (fig. 5). Differentiating between benign and malignant pathology is always more difficult in the case of lobular calcifications.

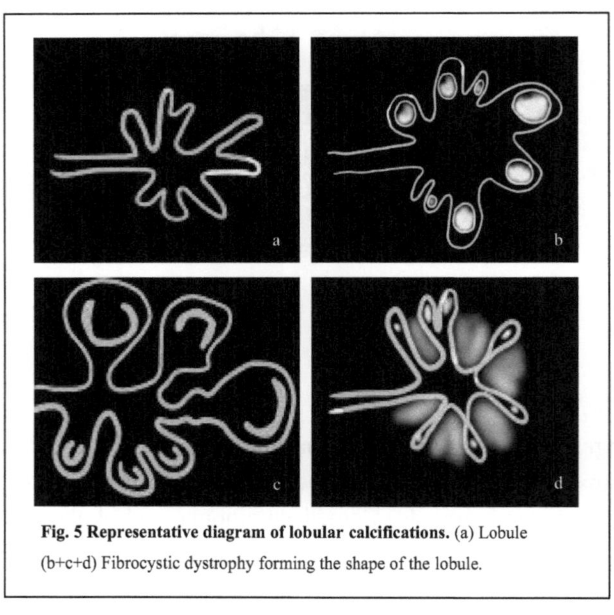

Fig. 5 Representative diagram of lobular calcifications. (a) Lobule (b+c+d) Fibrocystic dystrophy forming the shape of the lobule.

PHYSICOCHEMICAL REMINDER

Frappart has shown that there are two types of microcalcifications [2, 3], based on the study of breast exeresis specimens using light and electron microscopy (transmission and scanning), microanalysis and X-ray diffraction:

- type 1 calcium oxalate microcalcifications (Weddellite): These account for 10% of microcalcifications. These crystalline microcalcifications are amber in colour and almost transparent. Under light microscopy, they can go unnoticed with standard stains, but are highly birefringent under polarised light and are stained with alizarin red. On electron microscopy, they are polyhedral in shape, with a smooth surface and well-defined edges. These calcifications are benign in 95% of cases. In mammography, they sometimes take on a pathognomonic polyhedral shape, but most of the time these calcifications are perceived as round or oval images due to the "MACH" effect and the poor spatial resolution of mammography, which means that no practical conclusions can be drawn when interpreting mammograms;
- Type 2 calcium phosphate microcalcifications: These account for 90% of microcalcifications. Their structure is not crystalline; they are generally ovoid or fusiform. Under light microscopy, they are stained purple by haematein and are not birefringent under polarised light. Under electron microscopy, their surfaces are irregular, as they are formed by the coalescence of small spheres or oolites. These microcalcifications correspond to both malignant and benign pathologies [4].

MAMMOGRAPHY

1.Technical

Mammography is the benchmark radiological examination for screening for breast cancer, which is the leading cause of death in women.
Mammographic images must be optimised in terms of spatial resolution, contrast and noise. Several technical criteria must be taken into account, in particular, the contrast must be high in order to visualise microcalcifications properly. The radiation spectrum must be broad in order to adapt to the varying densities of the breasts and the minimum radiation dose, especially in young patients.

2.Positioning

Positioning the breast is a fundamental stage in mammography, and the technique must be beyond reproach. The aim is to radiograph the entire mammary gland, including the deep planes. Positioning is the key to obtaining images of optimum quality, which are essential for interpretation and meet a number of quality criteria [5].

2.1. Fundamental impacts

2.1.1. Front or cranio-caudal view

The X-ray beam approaches the breast craniocaudally (fig. 6).

Difficulty of frontal incidence

In the absence of visualization of the deep mammary planes, it is important to engage as much posterior mammary tissue as possible.
Good incidence criteria (fig. 7)

The breast is in the centre of the image. The gland is well spread out.

The nipple is at its zenith [6]. No folds or overlaps.
The pectoralis muscle is visible in almost 30% of cases, and its presence on the image allows optimum depth gain [5].

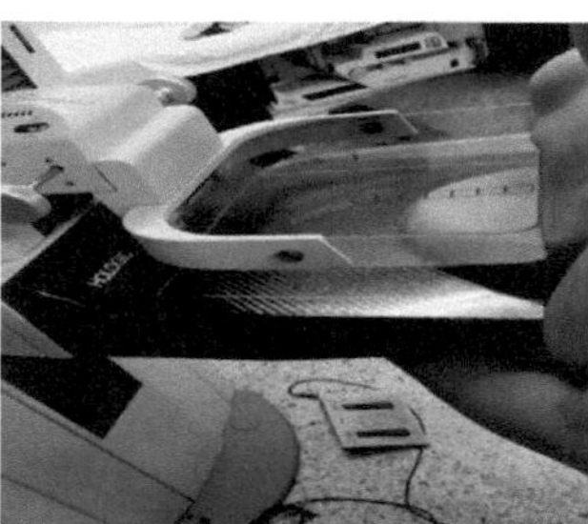

Fig. 6: Frontal or craniocaudal incision.

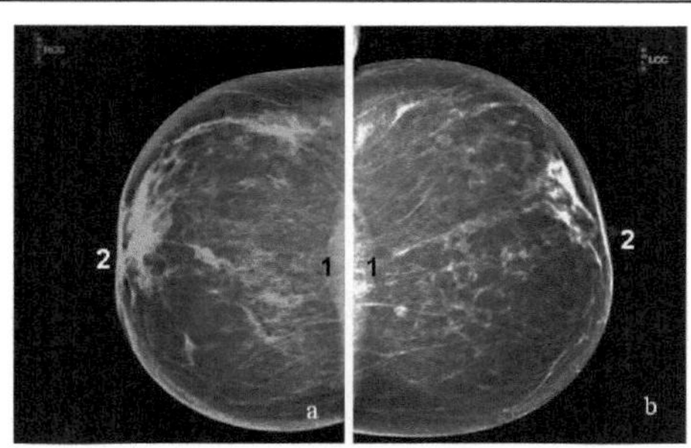

Fig. 7 Quality criteria for the frontal view. Mammographic images. (a) Right side. (b) Left side. Pectoral muscle (1), nipple at zenith (2).

2.1.2. 45° external oblique incidence°

This angle allows the breast to be studied in its long axis and a maximum amount of breast tissue to be analysed [7]. The stand is tilted at a strict 45° angle° , to ensure reproducible views (fig. 8).
Difficulty of oblique incidence

Compress the pectoral muscle, breast and submammary fold evenly.

Good incidence criteria (fig. 9)

The pectoral muscle is visible up to halfway up the image [8]. The nipple is at the zenith, opposite the tip of the pectoral muscle [7]. Presence of the skin fold of the abdominal wall [6].The long axis of the breast tends towards the horizontal.Presence of the "open" submammary fold, perfectly clear of the abdominal wall [9].No creases or overlapping.

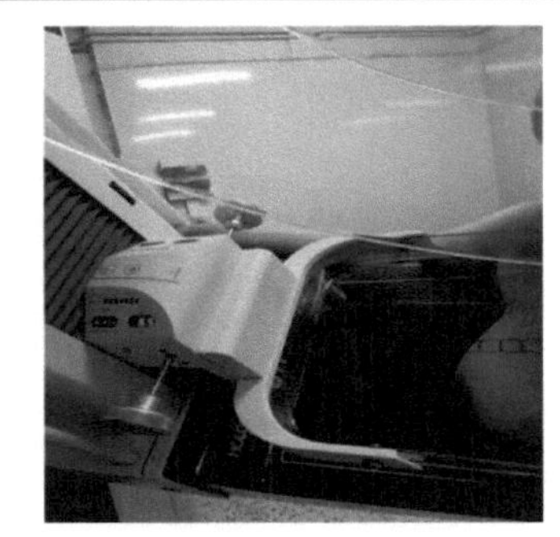

Fig. 8: External oblique incision.

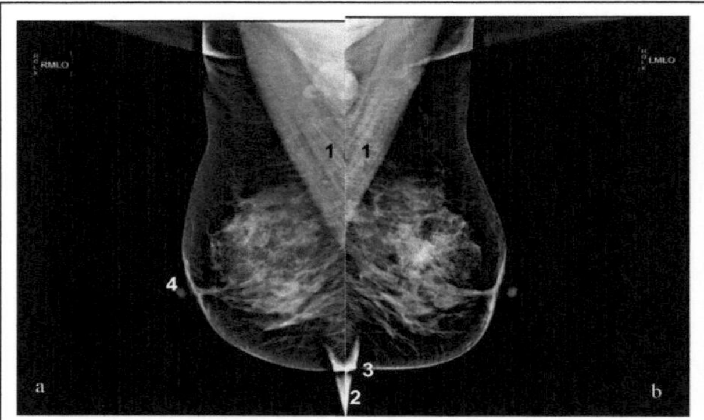

Fig. 9 Quality criteria for external oblique incidence. Mammographic images (a) Right oblique (b) Left oblique. Pectoral muscle (1), skin fold of the abdominal wall (2), open sub mammary fold (3),
nipple at the zenith (4).

2.2. Additional impacts

They are always carried out in addition to the fundamental impacts.

2.2.1. Profile incidence

It is useful for determining the precise location of a lesion. It can also be used to show whether microcalcifications are located in a horizontal position.

2.2.2. Centred localized image

It can be used to analyse the contours of a nodule or a stellar image, or to eliminate a constructed image (fig. 10).

2.2.3. Enlarged centred image

Microcalcifications visible on standard images can be enlarged for detailed analysis (number, appearance, organisation, etc.) (fig. 11).

2.3. Other impacts

Axillary extension, Cleopatra incidence, staggered frontal incidence, tangential view, Eklund manoeuvre [10-13].

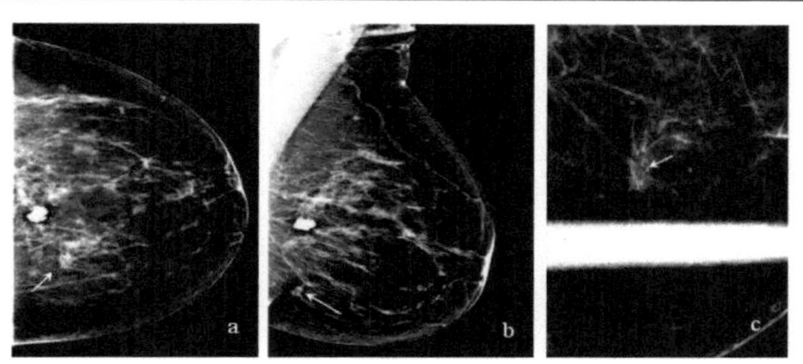

Fig. 10. Centred localized view. (a) Front view. Mass with indistinct contours (arrow). (b) External oblique view. Mass in the sub mammary fold with poorly defined contours (arrow). (c). Centred view located on the mass. Spiculated mass, BIRADS 5 (arrow).

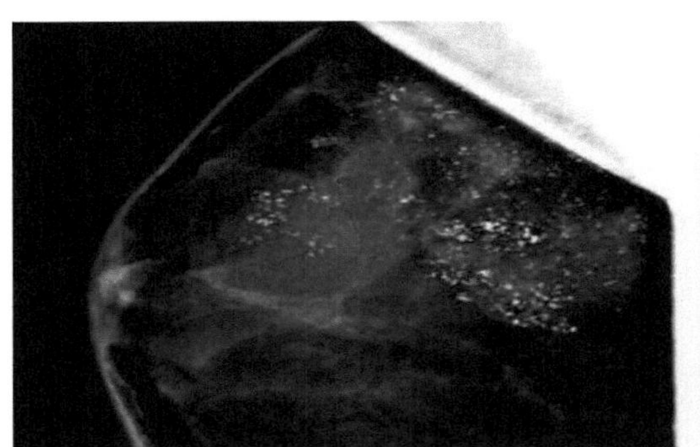

Fig. 11. Enlarged centred view. Magnification of a focus of micro-calcifications.

BI-RADS CALCIFICATION OF THE ACR

Mammographic images are currently interpreted according to the American College of Radiology (ACR) BI-RADS guidelines [14]. This standard provides a categorisation of all breast lesions, particularly microcalcifications. This classification has the advantage of being used by all breast specialists. It helps to limit inter-observer discrepancies, particularly with training. This classification takes into account the shape, but also more importantly the topography and distribution of the microcalcifications. This reference system is used to classify mammograms according to the ACR predictive classification, ranging from 0 to 6 (table 1).

Table 1. BI-RADS mammography assessment categories	
BI-RADS 0	Incomplete assessment requiring further imaging
BI-RADS 1	Normal mammography
BI-RADS 2	Benign abnormality.
BI-RADS 3	Anomaly probably benign, with a risk of malignancy < 2%, short-term monitoring is recommended.
BI-RADS 4	Suspicious abnormality, with a probability of malignancy of between 3% and 95%, requiring histological analysis. 4a = low probability, 4b = moderate probability, 4c = high probability.
BI-RADS 5	Highly suspicious abnormality, with a probability of malignancy > 95%, requiring surgical removal.
BI-RADS 6	Known histological result: proven malignancy.

BI-RADS GLOSSARY

The BI-RADS classification breaks down intramammary calcifications into two types, essentially taking into account their morphology and distribution: typically benign calcifications.suspicious calcifications. The degree of suspicion of malignancy is increased according to the distribution and size of the focus.

1.Morphology of calcifications

1.1. Typically benign calcifications

Benign calcifications, such as cystic "ring" calcifications, vascular calcifications, cutaneous calcifications, etc., are usually regular, smooth-edged, round if their size is between They are generally regular, with smooth edges, round if their size is between 0.5 and 1 mm and punctiform if their size is less than 0.5 mm.

1.1.1. Skin calcifications

Calcium deposits with a clear centre, often pathognomonic, they are usually seen along the submammary fold, in the paraspinal, axillary and areolar regions. In the case of unusual forms, tangential incidence can confirm their subcutaneous topography (fig. 12).

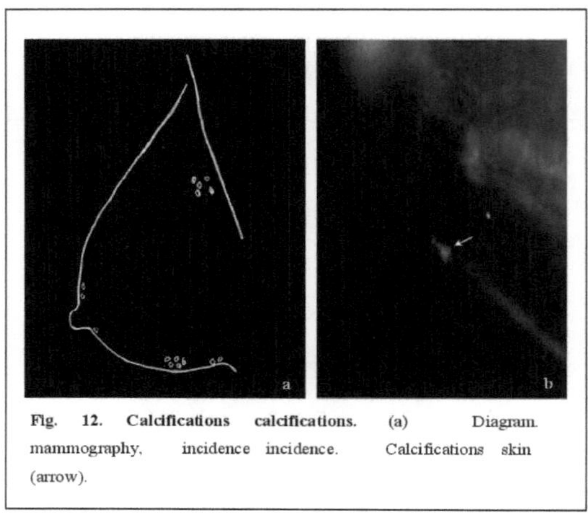

Fig. 12. Calcifications calcifications. (a) Diagram. mammography. incidence incidence. Calcifications skin (arrow).

1.1.2. Vascular calcifications

Rail or linear calcifications, clearly associated with tubular structures (fig. 13).

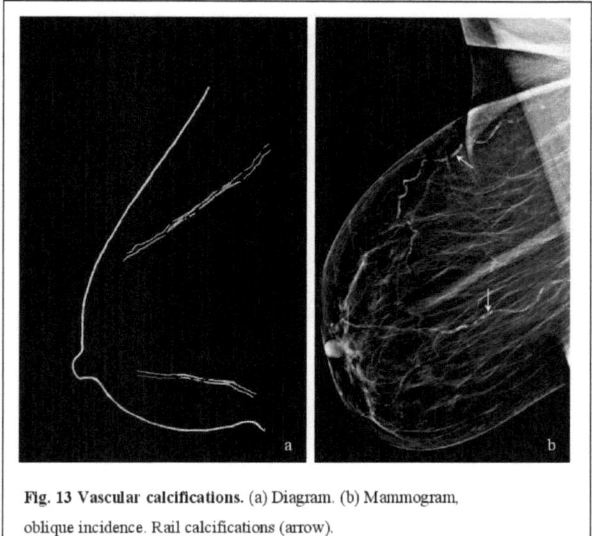

Fig. 13 Vascular calcifications. (a) Diagram. (b) Mammogram, oblique incidence. Rail calcifications (arrow).

1.1.3. Coarse or coralliform calcifications

These are large calcifications, greater than 2-3 mm in diameter, generally secondary to involution of a fibroadenoma (figs. 14, 15).

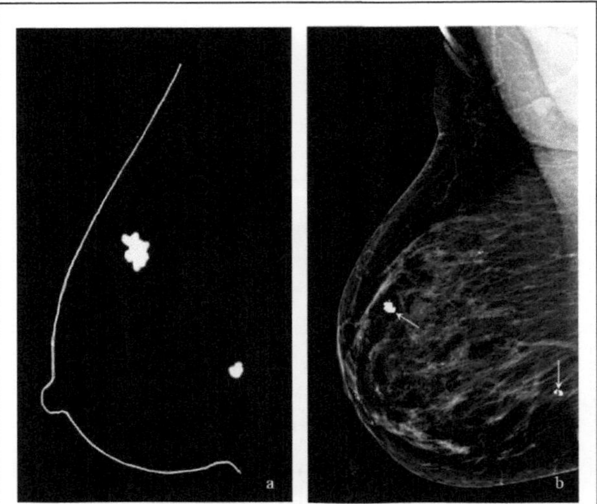

Fig. 14 Coralliform calcifications (a) Diagram. (b) Mammogram, oblique incidence. Large calcifications (arrows).

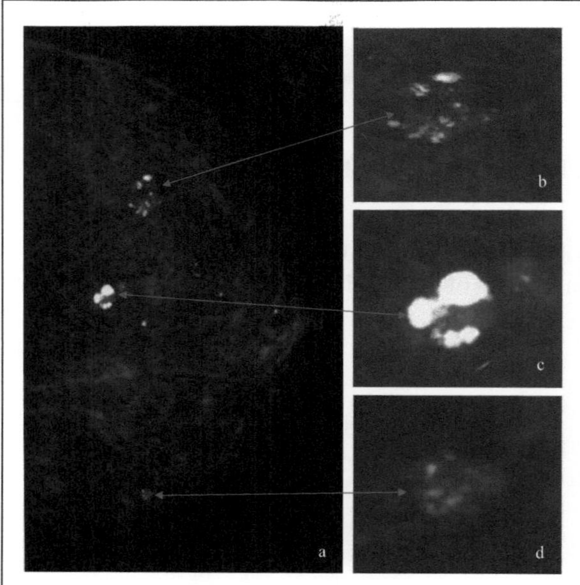

Fig. 15: Coralliform calcifications (a) Mammography, frontal view (b+c+d) Enlargements. Calcifications of fibroadenoma in the process of

1.1.4. Large rod calcifications

These are secretory calcifications associated with ductal ectasia which form smooth-edged rods, sometimes discontinuous, of supra-millimetre size. These calcifications may have a clear centre if the calcium is deposited in the wall of the galactophore (fig. 16). They are distributed along the nipple, usually bilaterally. They are often found in patients over 60 years of age.

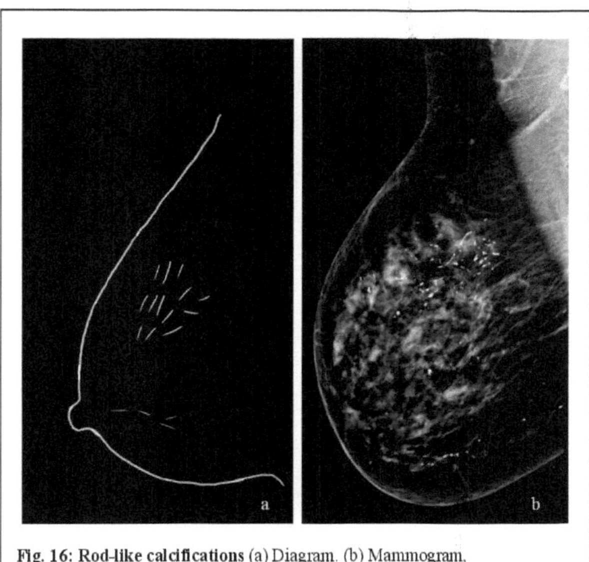

Fig. 16: Rod-like calcifications (a) Diagram. (b) Mammogram, oblique angle. Linear calcifications directed towards the nipple (arrows).

1.1.5. Round calcifications

Round calcifications are often multiple and vary in size. They are considered benign when they are scattered. When they are small, less than 1 mm, they frequently correspond to calcium deposits in the lobular acini (fig. 17). When they are less than 0.5 mm, the term punctiform is used. Usually benign, a cluster of microcalcifications is more suspicious and may need to be monitored if it has appeared, or if it is present on the same side as a breast cancer (fig. 18).

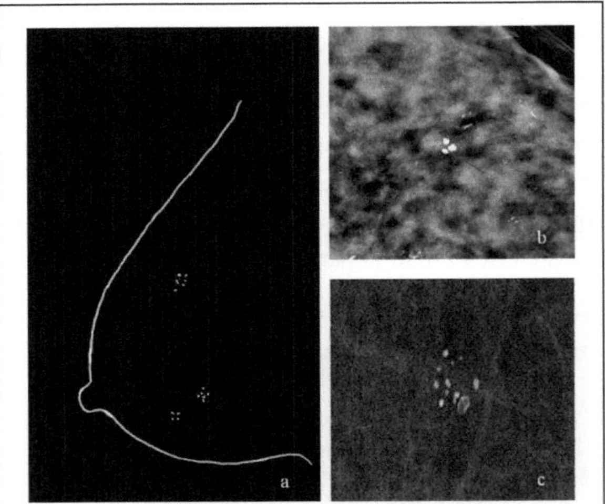

Fig. 17. round calcifications. (a) Diagram. (b+c) Mammogram. Clusters round calcifications (arrows).

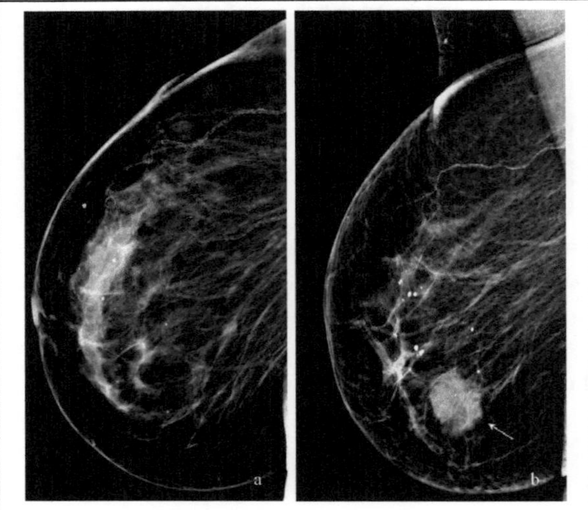

Fig. 18. round calcifications. (a+b) Mammogram. (a) Scattered round calcifications. (b) Round calcifications associated with a suspicious mass. (arrow).

1.1.6. Calcifications with a clear centre

Calcifications ranging in size from a millimetre to a centimetre, corresponding to calcifications of cytosteatonecrosis or calcified ductal debris. They are round or oval with a smooth surface and a clear centre with a thicker wall than eggshell calcifications (fig. 19).

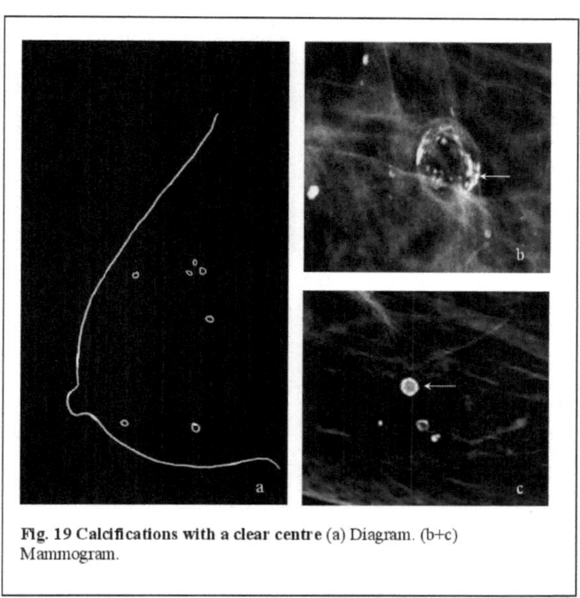

Fig. 19 Calcifications with a clear centre (a) Diagram. (b+c) Mammogram.

1.1.7. Eggshell" or parietal calcifications

These are very fine calcifications with the appearance ofa calcium deposit on the surface of a sphere. These deposits are very thin, generally less than 1 mm thick.)

The two main etiologies are :

- calcification of the cyst walls (fig. 20);

- cytosteatonecrosis (fig. 21).

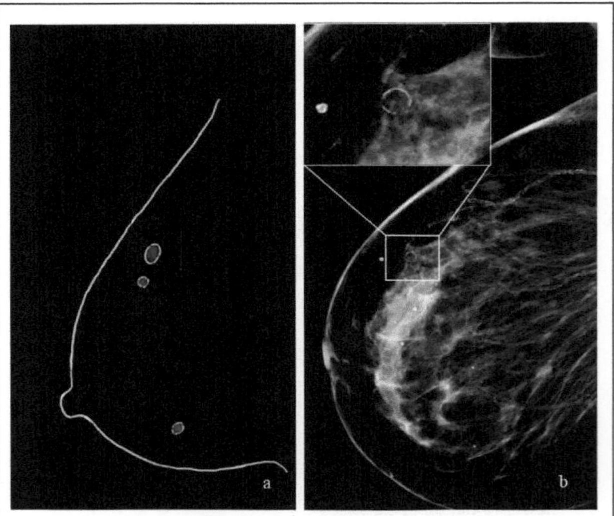

Fig. 20 Eggshell calcifications (a) Diagram. (b) Mammogram. Calcifications with calcium deposits on the surface of a cystic wall.

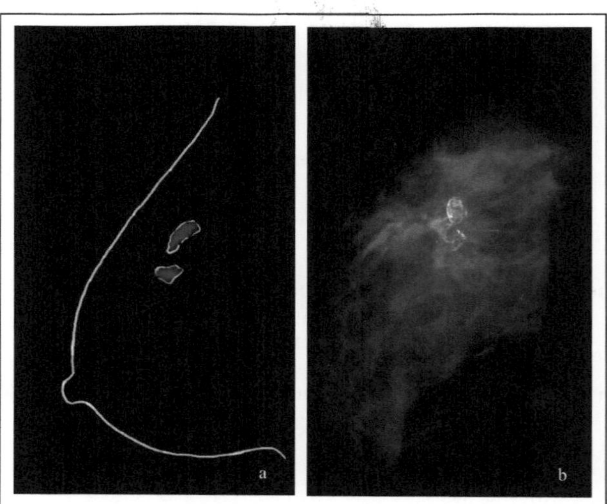

Fig. 21 Eggshell calcifications (a) Diagram. (b) Mammogram. Calcifications with a depositcalcium on the surface of a lesion of cytosteatonecrosis (arrows).

1.1.8. Calcium milk-type calcifications

They are secondary to intracystic sedimentation of calcified secretion products. On mammographic views from the front, they appear as amorphous deposits with blurred boundaries. On the strict profile, however, they are clear, semilunar, crescent-shaped or curvilinear with an upper concavity, or linear, forming the sloping part of the cysts (fig. 22).

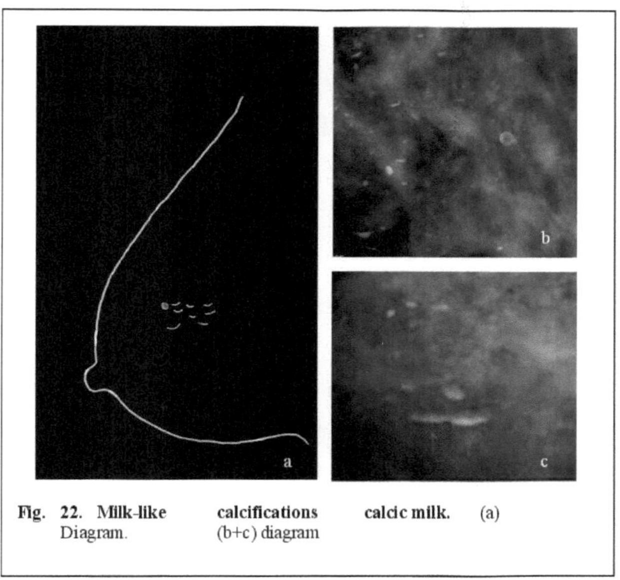

Fig. 22. Milk-like calcifications calcic milk. (a) Diagram. (b+c) diagram

1.1.9. Calcified sutures

These calcifications correspond to calcium deposits on suture material. They are more frequent in the irradiated breast. They appear as linear calcifications following the path of the sutures (fig. 23).

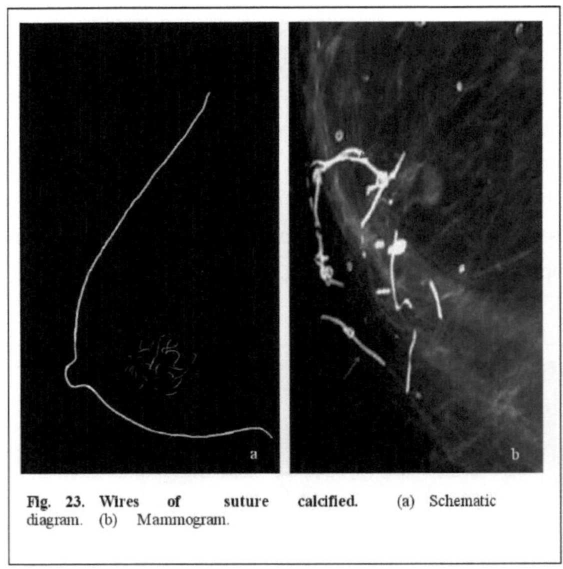

Fig. 23. Wires of suture calcified. (a) Schematic diagram. (b) Mammogram.

1.1.10. Dystrophic calcifications

These calcifications usually appear in irradiated breasts or after breast trauma. They are often irregular in shape, coarse and supramillimetric (fig. 24).

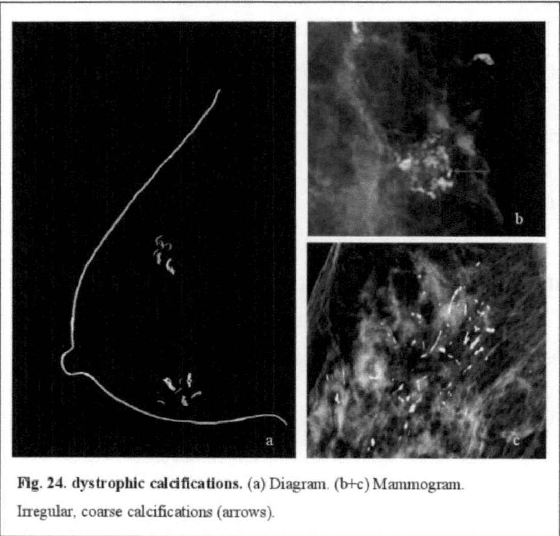

Fig. 24. dystrophic calcifications. (a) Diagram. (b+c) Mammogram. Irregular, coarse calcifications (arrows).

1.2. Calcifications suspected of being malignant

Four terms from the lexicon can be described: amorphous calcifications, coarse and heterogeneous calcifications, polymorphic fine calcifications and linear fine calcifications or branches.

1.2.1. Amorphous microcalcifications

These are very fine calcifications, making it impossible to determine a specific form. When these calcifications are organised in isolated foci, they must be classified in the BI-RADS 4b category (10-50% malignancy), with a positive predictive value (PPV) of malignancy of 20% (fig. 25). The diffuse distribution of these microcalcifications may be benign.

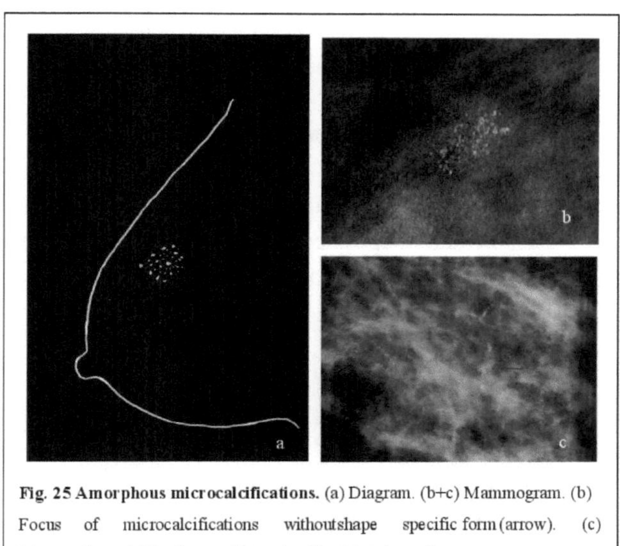

Fig. 25 Amorphous microcalcifications. (a) Diagram. (b+c) Mammogram. (b) Focus of microcalcifications withoutshape specific form (arrow). (c) Linear microcalcifications, with no specific shape (arrow).

1.2.2. Coarse, heterogeneous microcalcifications

They are irregular calcifications more often organised in clusters, between 0.5 and 1 mm in size, and by definition smaller than dystrophic calcifications (> 1 mm) (fig. 26). They may be malignant or benign and are seen in fibroadenomas or cytosteonecrosis. In the case of an isolated focus of microcalcifications, they should be classified as BI-RADS 4b, with a PPV of malignancy of 15%.

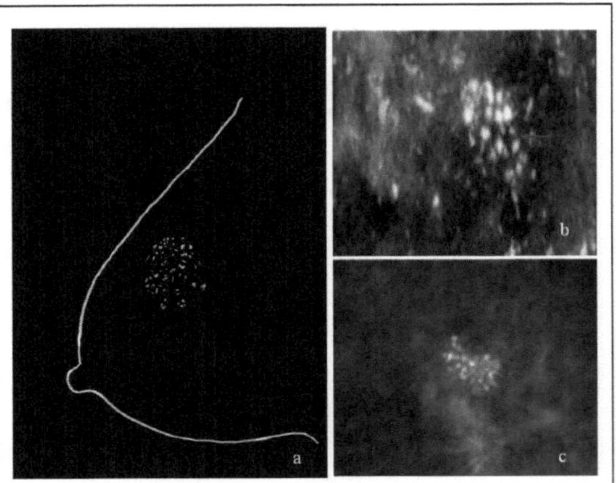

Fig. 26: Coarse, heterogeneous microcalcifications (a) Diagram. (b+c) Mammogram. (b) Focal area of microcalcifications (arrow): non-specific infiltrating carcinoma (arrow). (c) Focus of microcalcifications: fibroadenoma. (arrow).

1.2.3. Fine polymorphic microcalcifications

They are generally more visible than amorphous calcifications, with no linear path (fig. 27). Their size and shape are irregular and variable, but usually less than 0.5 mm. They should be classified as BI-RADS 4b, with a PPV of 29%.

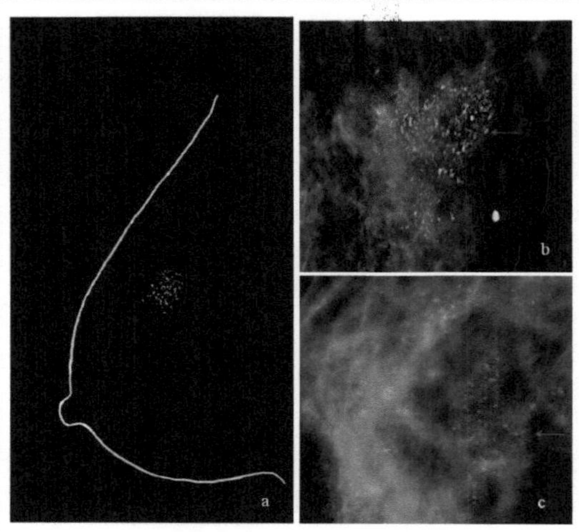

Fig. 27. Fine, polymorphic microcalcifications. (a) Diagram. (b+c) Mammography. Microcalcifications polymorphous, irregular (arrow): non-specific infiltrating carcinoma.

1.2.4. Fine linear or branched calcifications

They are generally linear or irregularly curved and less than 0.5 mm in size (fig. 28). Their morphology is suggestive of the filling of a galactophore duct by tumour necrosis. They have a very high PPV of malignancy (70%) and, whatever their distribution, must be classified as at least BI-RADS 4c.

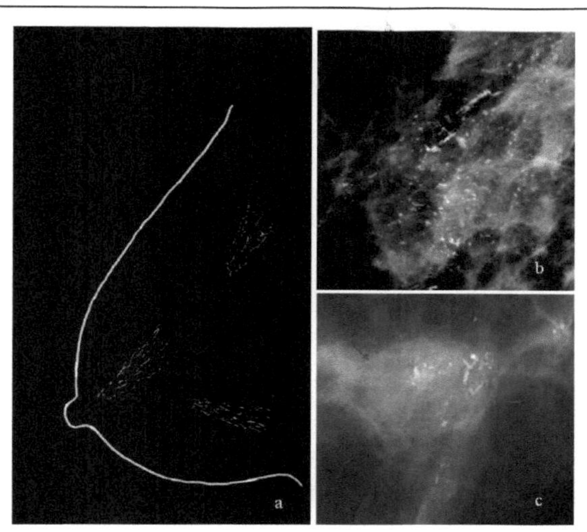

Fig. 28. Linear or branched fine calcifications. (a) Diagram. (b+c) Mammogram. Fine linear branching calcifications. (c) Irregular, spiculated mass associated with microcalcifications (arrows): infiltrating carcinoma of non-specific type.

2.Distribution of calcifications

The distribution of microcalcifications must also be analysed. There are five types of distribution: diffuse, regional, clustered, linear and segmental.

2.1. Diffuse distribution

These are calcifications distributed randomly and sparsely in the breast, and are generally benign (fig. 29).

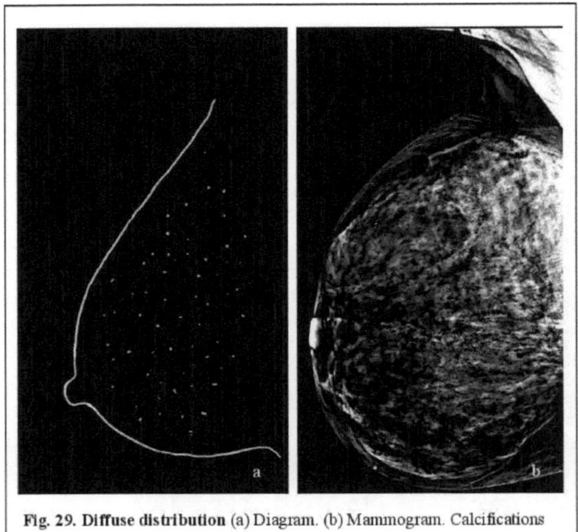

Fig. 29. Diffuse distribution (a) Diagram. (b) Mammogram. Calcifications scattered.

2.2. Regional distribution

These are calcifications grouped together in a volume over 2 cm in diameter, but with no galactophoric orientation (fig. 30).

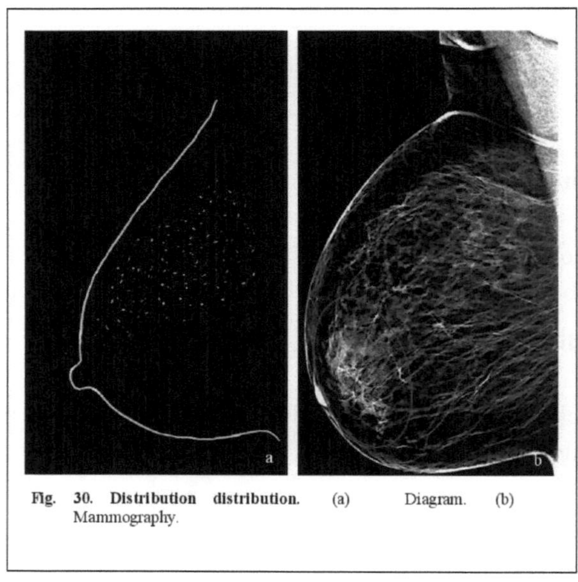

Fig. 30. Distribution distribution. (a) Diagram. (b) Mammography.

2.3. Group distribution

They correspond to a grouping of at least five microcalcifications within 1 cm and less than 2 cm (fig. 31).

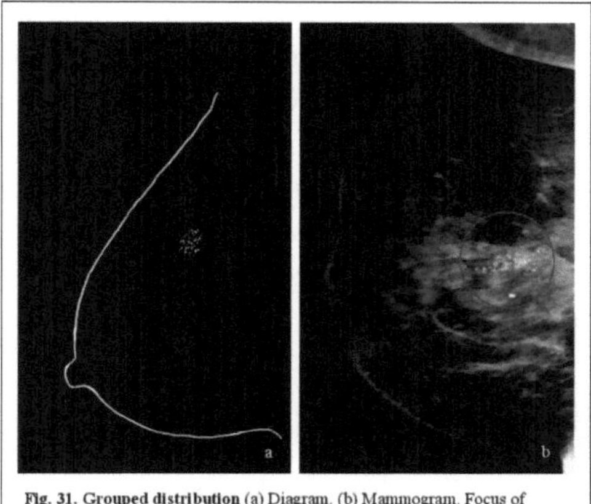

Fig. 31. Grouped distribution (a) Diagram. (b) Mammogram. Focus of microcalcifications extending over 2 cm (circle).

2.4. Linear distribution

These are calcifications with a galactophoric, linear course (fig. 32). This distribution is suggestive of intra-galactophoreal calcium deposits and its presence increases the suspicion of malignancy.

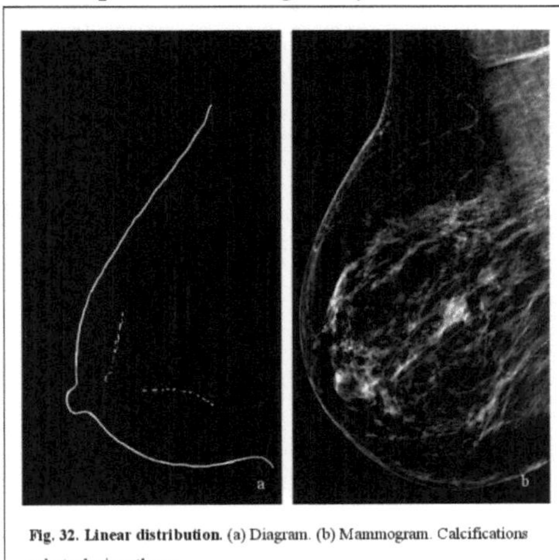

Fig. 32. Linear distribution. (a) Diagram. (b) Mammogram. Calcifications galactophoric pathway.

2.5. Segmented distribution

The calcifications are triangular in distribution, with a peripheral base and apex converging towards the nipple (fig. 33).

Segmentally distributed calcifications are worrying because they suggest calcium deposits in the milk ducts, raising the possibility of extensive or multifocal breast carcinoma in a lobe or segment of the breast.Benign segmental calcifications, such as secretory calcifications, exist. Their smooth rod morphology and large size generally make it possible to differentiate benign calcifications of galactophoric ectasia from the finer, more irregular malignant calcifications of intra-canal carcinomas. A segmental distribution greatly increases the degree of suspicion for punctiform or amorphous calcifications and requires histological examination.

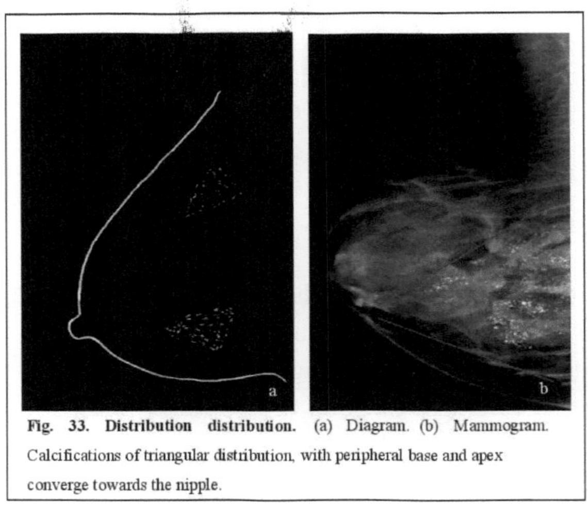

Fig. 33. Distribution distribution. (a) Diagram. (b) Mammogram. Calcifications of triangular distribution, with peripheral base and apex converge towards the nipple.

The positive predictive values (PPV) of malignancy associated with microcalcifications according to their morphology and distribution are summarised in Table 2.

Table 2.Predictive values of malignancy associatedmicrocalcifications according to their morphology and distribution according to BI-RADS 2013.			
Calcifications Distribution Morphology	Diffuse (VPP = 0)	Regional, grouped (PPV: 26-31%)	Linear, segmental (PPV: 60-68%)
Round or punctiform	BI-RADS 2	BI-RADS 3	BI-RADS 4a
Heterogeneous coarse	BI-RADS 2	BI-RADS 4b	BI-RADS 4c
Amorphous or pleiomorphous	BI-RADS 2/3	BI-RADS 4b	BI-RADS 4c
Linear	BI-RADS 4a	BI-RADS 4c	BI-RADS 5

ACR BI-RADS MAMMOGRAPHY CLASSIFICATION

The ACR BI-RADS classification is summarised in table 3 [14].

Table 3. Classification of mammographic abnormalities

BI-RADS	ACR BI-RADS classification Mammography and treatment guidelines (CAT)
BI-RADS 0	Mammography pending further diagnosis
BI-RADS 1	Normal mammography
BI-RADS 2	Abnormalities considered benign (PPV of cancer = 0%). Skin and vascular calcifications. Large, light-centred, parietal, milk-calcium calcifications, dystrophic, calcified sutures. Diffuse regular round calcifications.
BI-RADS 3	Anomalies considered probably benign (PPV of cancer < 2%) CAT: short-term monitoring 4 to 6 months recommended Round or amorphous calcifications, few in number and in small isolated round clusters. Small, round or oval cluster of polymorphous calcifications, with littlenumerous, suggesting the onset of calcification of an adenofibroma.
BI-RADS 4	Anomalies considered suspicious (PPV > 2% and < 95%) CAT: biopsy. Numerous round calcifications and/or clusters of calcifications that are neither round nor oval in shape. Calcifications amorphous or dusty, grouped and numerous. Calcifications coarse heterogeneous or fine calcifications few polymorphs.
BI-RADS 5	Abnormalities considered to be malignant (PPV > 95%) CAT: biopsy and multidisciplinary management. Fine linear or fine linear, branched calcifications. Coarse heterogeneous calcifications or fine polymorphic calcifications, numerous and grouped in clusters. Grouped calcifications of any morphology, with linear or segmental distribution (intragalactophoric topography). Calcifications associated with architectural distortion or a mass.Grouped calcifications that have increased in number or calcifications whose morphology and distribution have become more suspect.
BI-RADS 6	Known cancer, malignancy proven by biopsy CAT: biopsy and multidisciplinary management.

MAMMARY CALCIFICATIONS AND PATHOLOGIES

The BI-RADS classification looks at the risk of malignancy as a function of the morphology and distribution of breast calcifications, providing practical guidelines for action, but without systematically addressing breast pathology. Another way of approaching breast calcifications is to study the shape of the calcifications in relation to the breast pathology, which allows a more systematic study of breast microcalcifications.

1.Benign breast diseases and calcifications

1.1. Superficial calcifications

They correspond to calcifications of the subcutaneous plane. There are three main types (fig. 34):
- Calcifications of the sebaceous glands;
- scarring calcifications ;
- calcific microcystic lipo necrosis.

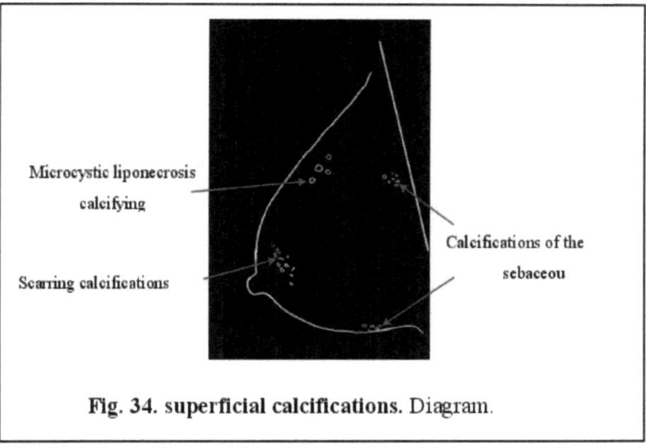

Fig. 34. superficial calcifications. Diagram.

1.1.1. Calcifications of the sebaceous glands

These are calcifications of the sweat glands. They generally take the form of multiple, fairly dense, rounded or polygonal calcifications, with transparent or umbilicated centres (fig. 35). They are between 1 and 2 mm in size. They are most often found along the sub mammary fold, in the axillary, parasternal and areolar regions. Mammographic views of the face and oblique are sometimes insufficient to confirm that they are intra-dermal. It is essential to take a tangential film to confirm that they are subcutaneous. These are benign calcifications classified as BI-RADS 2 by the ACR.

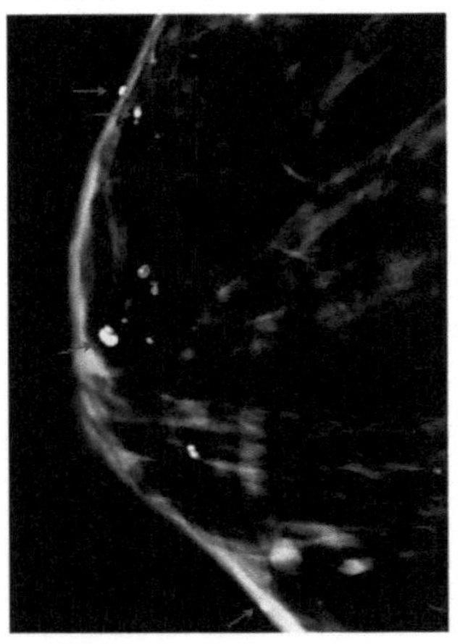

Fig. 35. Calcifications of the sebaceous glands. Mammogram. Calcifications of the periareolar sebaceous glands (arrows).

1.1.2. Scarring calcifications

These calcifications are quite similar to the calcifications of the sebaceous glands. They correspond to round or polyhedral calcifications with a clear centre, between 1 and 2 mm in size (fig. 36). They differ from sebaceous gland calcifications in that they are more monomorphic and not grouped in clusters. They are most often found in the periareolar area secondary to surgery, or at the union of the lower quadrants, in the sub mammary fold.

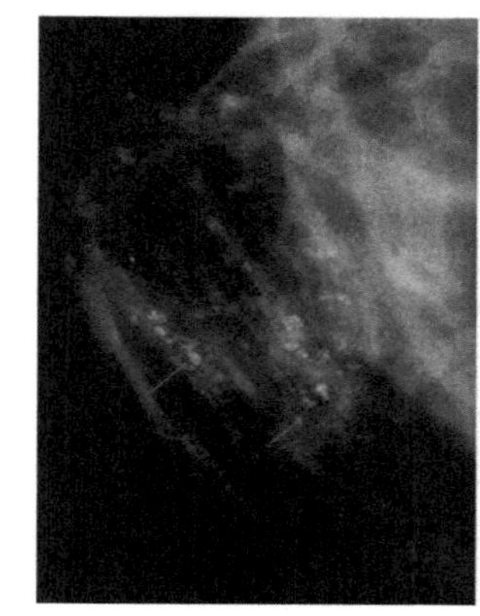

Fig. 36. Calcifications scarring. Mammography. Round, polyhedral, periareolar calcifications, some with light centre (arrows) [15].

1.1.3. Calcific microcystic liponecrosis

This is a particular form of cytosteatonecrosis associated with repeated micro-trauma, particularly in patients with large breasts. They correspond to calcifications with a clear centre, larger than other superficial calcifications (fig. 37). They are located in the hypodermis.

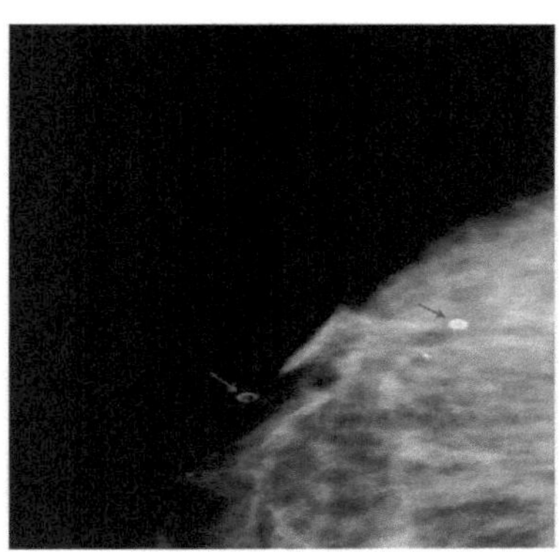

Fig. 37. Calcific microcystic liponecrosis. Mammogram. Superficial calcifications with clear centres (arrows).

1.2. Vascular calcifications

These are calcifications located in the wall of the mammary arteries. They are linked to systemic atherosclerosis or disorders of phosphocalcic metabolism. They are present in 10% of mammograms. Their frequency increases with age in people with diabetes or kidney failure. They are exceptional before the age of 50, even in cases of diabetes or renal failure. Most of the time, they appear on mammography as typical mural calcifications, arranged in parallel traces, partly linear and partly in patches along the vascular walls (fig. 38). They have a tortuous or serpentine configuration (fig. 38). When they are limited to a short segment, they may take on a linear or even canal-like appearance.

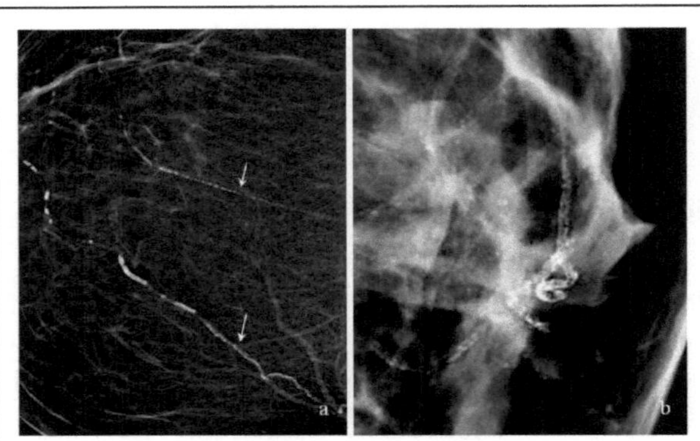

Fig. 38. Vascular calcifications. (a+b) Mammography: (a) Linear vascular calcifications (white arrows), plaques (red arrows). (b) Serpiginous vascular calcifications (red arrow).

1.3. Sequelae of galactophoritis calcifications

Secretory ductal ectasia is a benign inflammatory disease of the milk ducts, the next stage of which is represented by plasma cell mastitis. It corresponds to dilatation of the main milk ducts. This dilation is sometimes diffuse, but more often localised to the juxta-areolar region. It can be linked to the physiological development of the breast, which explains why it is so common in older women. At the beginning of the evolution, there is a simple dilatation and canal ectasia. At a later stage, there may be a peri-ductal inflammatory reaction. If this is moderate, the disease slowly progresses to fibrosis. On the other hand, if the inflammation is intense, it causes a rupture of the galactophore with extravasation of secretion products through the wall of the galactophore, which evolves into plasma cell mastitis with a reactive lymphoplasmacytic infiltrate. Sequelae of galactophoritis, which correspond to the rod-shaped calcifications of the BI-RADS classification, generally have an easily recognisable appearance, and may exist even in the absence of clinical signs. They are secondary to two different phenomena which affect the radiological image:

- calcification of the amorphous secretion products occupying the dilated duct. These calcifications take on a smooth, regular and rectilinear "broken needle" appearance (fig. 39). They may take on a more sinuous appearance with tapered ends."(fig. 40) ;

- perianal calcification due to extravasation of secretory products through the galactophore, which has become permeable as a result of the inflammatory process. When these calcifications are perilobular, they may take the form of non-specific "calcified microcysts" and when they are perichannel, they give "tubular calcifications with a clear centre" (figs 41, 42).

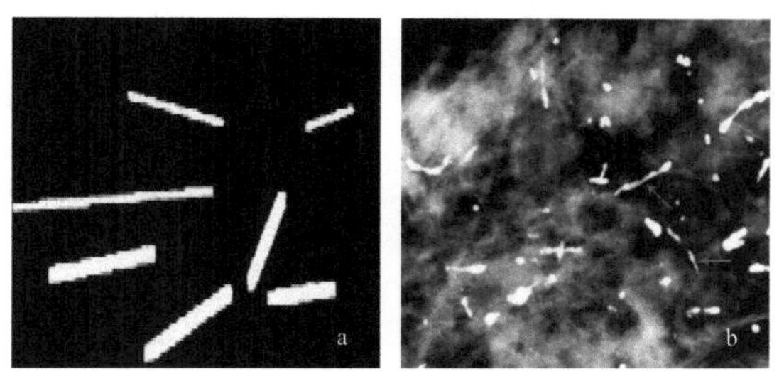

Fig. 39. Intracanal calcifications in broken needle. (a) Diagram. (b) Mammogram. Smooth, regular, straight calcifications (arrows).

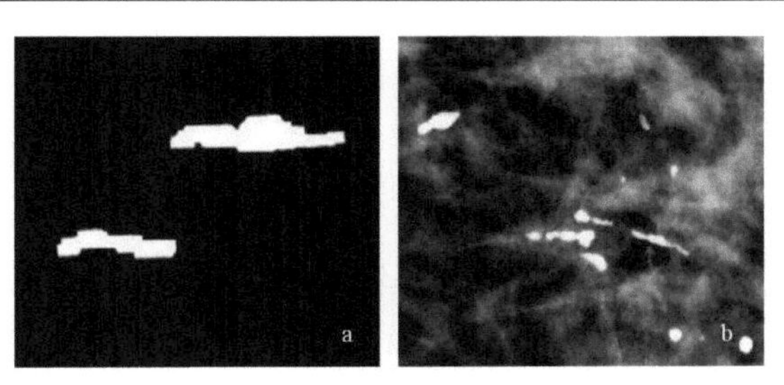

Fig. 40. Intracanal calcifications in barley s u g a r (a) Diagram. (b) Mammogram. Slightly sinuous calcifications with tapering ends (arrows).

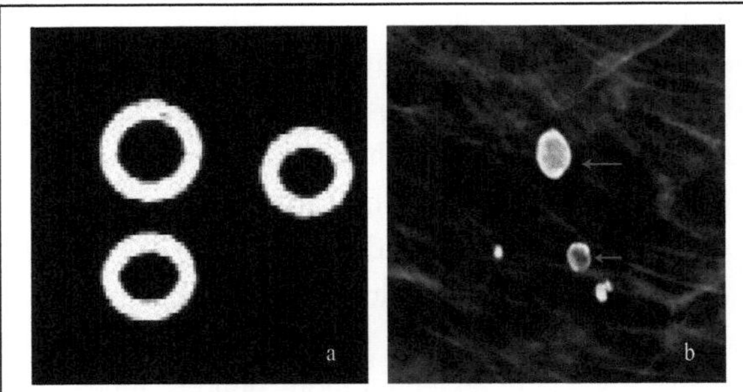

Fig. 41. Peri-lobular calcifications. (a) Diagram. (b) Mammogram. Calcified microcysts (arrows).

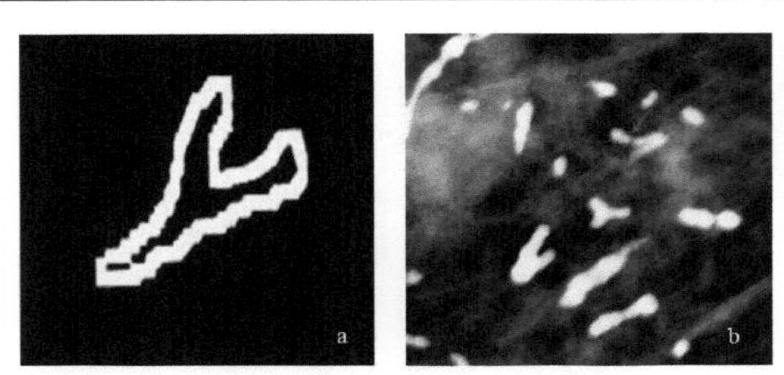

Fig. 42. Pericanal calcifications. (a) Diagram. (b) Mammogram. Tubular calcifications with clear centres (arrow).

1.4. Cytosteatonecrosis

Cytosteonecrosis corresponds to the necrosis of a fatty island of breast tissue which calcifies secondarily. This necrosis is either traumatic or iatrogenic (post-operative).

Typical forms do not generally pose any diagnostic problems:

- microcystic liponecrosis (fig. 37);
- eggshell calcifications (fig. 21, 43);
- calcifications with clear centres (fig. 43).

On the other hand, cytosteatonecrosis following surgery can pose diagnostic problems, particularly in the early stages, as the appearance of microcalcifications after cancer removal is a sign of recurrence in half of cases. It is the development of these microcalcifications that enables the diagnosis to be made.

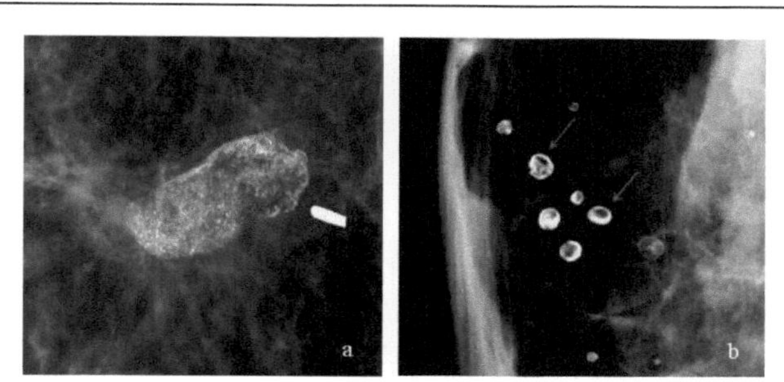

Fig. 43. Calcified cytosteatonecrosis. Mammography (a) Calcification in (b) Round calcifications with clear centres (arrows).

1.5. Fibroadenoma

Fibroadenoma is the benign fibro-epithelial tumour most frequently associated with calcifications. It is a lesion in young women, aged between 15 and 35, which develops at the expense of the ductulo-lobular unit with double epithelial and connective proliferation.

Clinically, fibroadenomas appear as a palpable mass that is generally painless, mobile, firm in consistency and variable in volume. They involute after the menopause and tend to calcify. They may be single, multiple or bilateral.

On mammography, they appear as a circumscribed, oval, rounded, lobulated mass, hypo- or isodense to the breast parenchyma. During the involution phase, this mass calcifies from the periphery towards the centre, taking on the typical appearance of coralliform calcifications (fig. 44). Sometimes the diagnosis is more difficult because the calcifications may take the form of coarse heterogeneous calcifications simulating a malignant lesion (fig. 45).

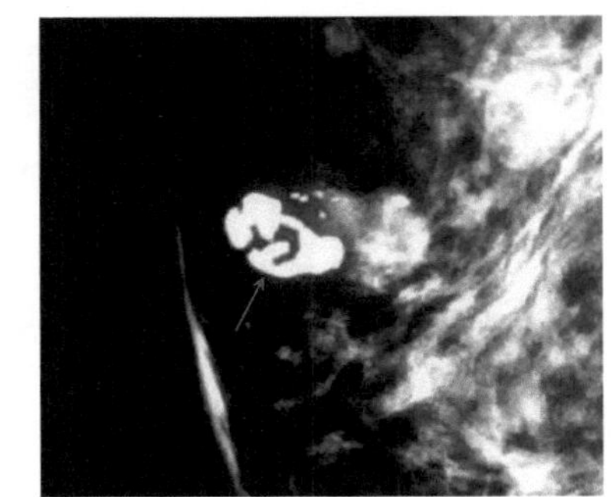

Fig. 44. Partially calcified fibroadenoma .
Mammogram. Mass showing coralliform calcification (arrow).

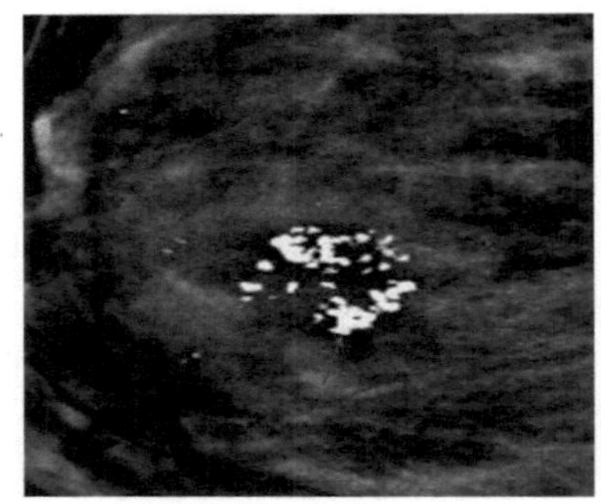

Fig. 45. Partially calcified fibroadenoma. Mammogram.
Heterogeneous, coarse calcifications (arrow).

1.6. Fibrocystic dystrophy

Fibrocystic disease encompasses a number of pathologies affecting both the epithelium of the galactophore and the surrounding connective tissue. Fibrocystic dystrophy is manifested by five histological lesions which explain the genesis and form of the microcalcifications encountered in this pathological entity: fibrosis, cystic hyperplasia, adenosis, apocrine metaplasia and epithelial hyperplasia.

1.6.1. Fibrosis

Fibrosis is a normal part of breast ageing. It affects, to varying degrees, the intra-lobular connective tissue and the extra-lobular connective tissue. This leads either to atrophy with the disappearance of the lobules and ducts, or to stricture of the galactophores leading to the formation of cysts in which calcium secretions settle (fig. 46).

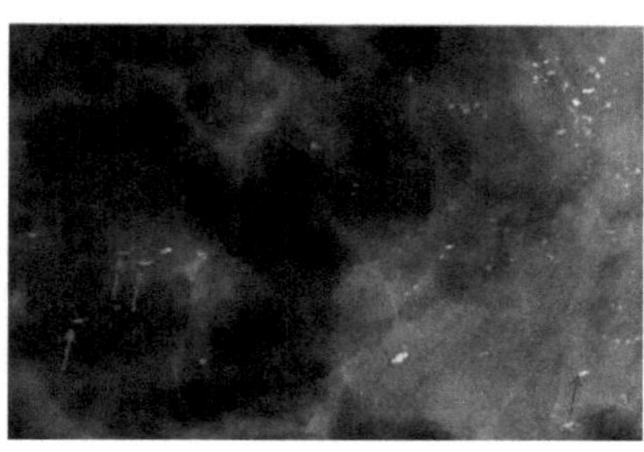

Fig. 46. Fibrosis. Mammogram. Calcifications secondary to sedimentation of calcium secretions (arrows).

1.6.2. Cystic hyperplasia

The formation of cysts is partly linked to fibrosis of the connective tissue, and partly to abnormalities in secretion and reabsorption in the galactophore duct, leading to stasis and upstream dilatation which encourages sedimentation. Cystic hyperplasia calcifications sometimes develop in the cyst in sedimentary form (calcifications of the milk-calcium type) or in the cyst walls (calcified microcysts) (fig. 47).

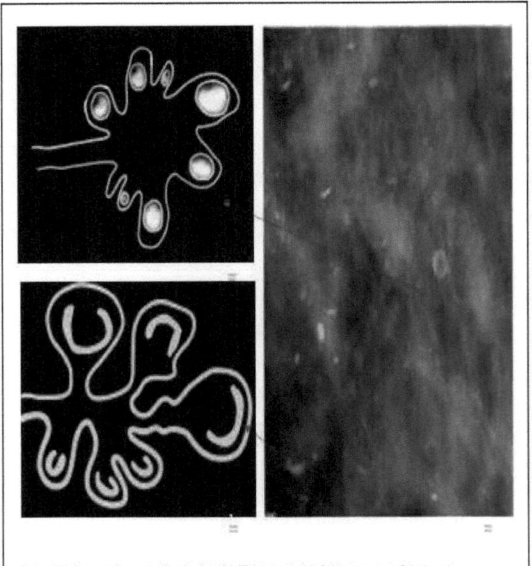

Fig. 47. Cystic hyperplasia (a+b) Diagram. (c) Mammography (a+c). Calcified micro-cyst. (b+c) Sedimentary calcifications

1.6.3. Adenosis

Adenosis is an increase in the number and size of lobules with proliferation of epithelial cells, myoepithelial cells and mantle connective tissue, promoting sedimentation of calcium salts in the acini of the UDTL. Adenosis calcifications are typically small, rounded calcifications, shaped like small pearls, grouped together in clusters in the shape of the acini of the UDTL. These calcifications are known as calcospherites (fig. 48). Sclerosing adenosis corresponds to the same phenomenon, with the addition of fibrosis of the peri-lobular connective tissue leading to a restriction and therefore a reduction in the size of the acini. The calcifications obtained are of the lobular type, varying in size and sometimes powdery (fig. 49).

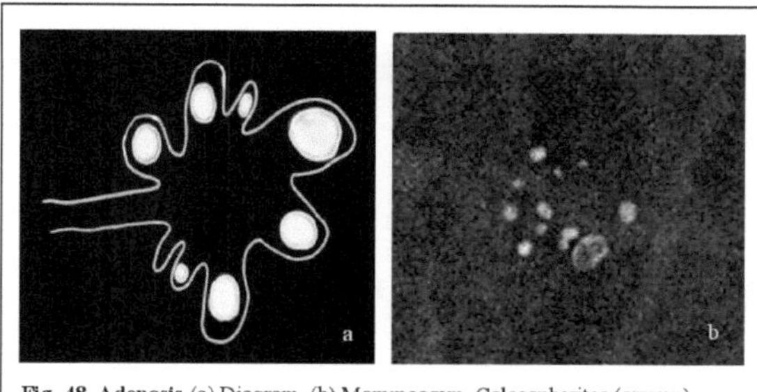

Fig. 48. Adenosis (a) Diagram. (b) Mammogram. Calcospherites (arrows).

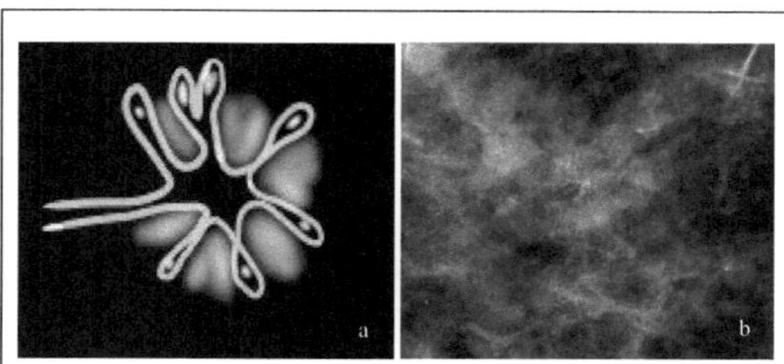

Fig. 49. Sclerosing adenosis (a) Diagram. (b) Mammogram. Focus of dusty microcalcifications (arrows).

1.6.4. Apocrine metaplasia

This is a transformation of the normal epithelium into a sweat epithelium, leading to an increase in the capacity to secrete calcium salts and a decrease in the capacity to reabsorb them, favouring the stasis of calcium secretions.

1.7. Simple epithelial hyperplasia

This is a benign proliferation of the glandular epithelium without cellular atypia. It is associated with an increase in the relative risk of breast cancer of 1.5 to 2. It is present in around 30% of breast biopsies. Clinically, simple epithelial hyperplasia is often asymptomatic, discovered by chance during a mammographic examination. It may be associated with other pathologies, such as ductal carcinoma in situ or infiltrating carcinoma.... On mammography, epithelial hyperplasia is usually not visible on the mammogram. It may show up as architectural disorganisation or foci of microcalcifications.

The microcalcification sites encountered are of all types, non-specific, but generally dusty, rounded or polymorphic microcalcifications.

1.8. Various calcifications

1.8.1. Calcifications of post-operative material

They correspond to calcifications of the suture material or, exceptionally, to calcifications of the compress, known as textiloma (fig. 50).

1.8.2. Parasitic calcifications

Filaria can cause mammary calcifications, reflecting their fossilisation. This condition, which is very common in Africa, is caused by Wuschiera Bancrofti. They may remain in the subcutaneous tissue, where they take on the characteristic appearance of serpiginous calcification (fig. 51). Occasionally, they may migrate into a galactophore, giving a misleading appearance. If there is any doubt, an X-ray of the hands, the most common site for filaria, should be carried out, as this will help to correct the diagnosis.
Other parasites can cause intramammary macrocalcifications, notably hydatosis, Medina filaria (Dracunculiasis) and Schisostomiasis.

1.8.3. Calcifications due to injected products

- related to silicone or paraffin injections;

- linked to the injection of lipiodol, a contrast agent used to produce galactograms.

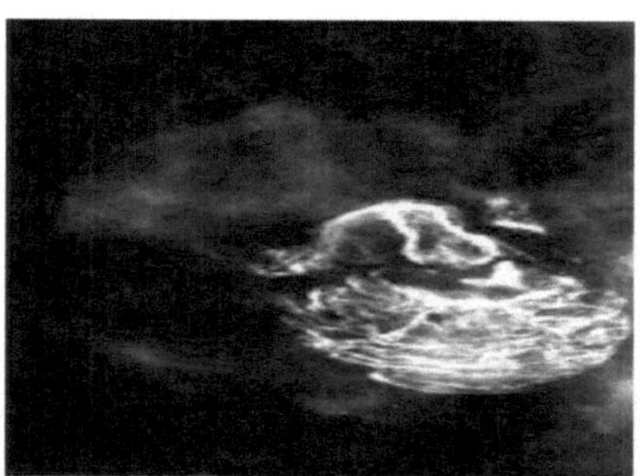

Fig. 50. Textilome. Mammogram. Calcified compress [15].

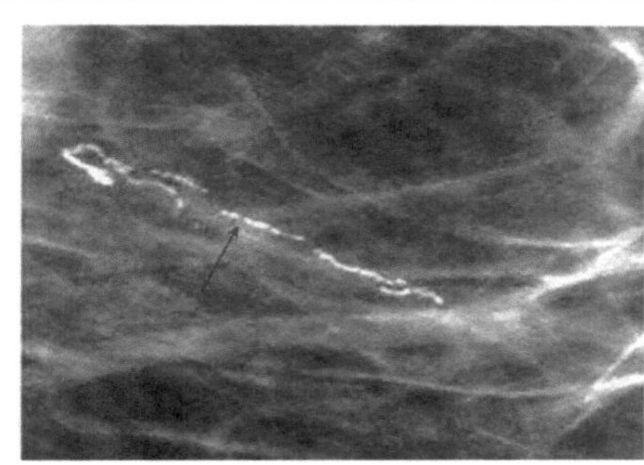

Fig. 51. Calcification parasitic calcification. Mammogram. Serpiginous calcification of mammary

2.Lesions at risk and calcifications

2.1. Atypical ductal hyperplasia

Atypical ductal hyperplasia is a proliferation of ductal glandular epithelium with cellular atypia. A lesion with a high risk of malignant degeneration, the relative risk of breast cancer is multiplied by 5 compared with the general population and multiplied by 11 in women with a first-degree family history.These lesions are generally asymptomatic. In rare cases, they may manifest as palpable masses. These lesions are often discovered histologically when a biopsy is taken in the presence of mammographic abnormalities. Mammography of atypical ductal hyperplasia is not specific. All types of amorphous, polymorphic, punctiform or rounded microcalcifications, masses and architectural disorganisation are found (fig. 52).

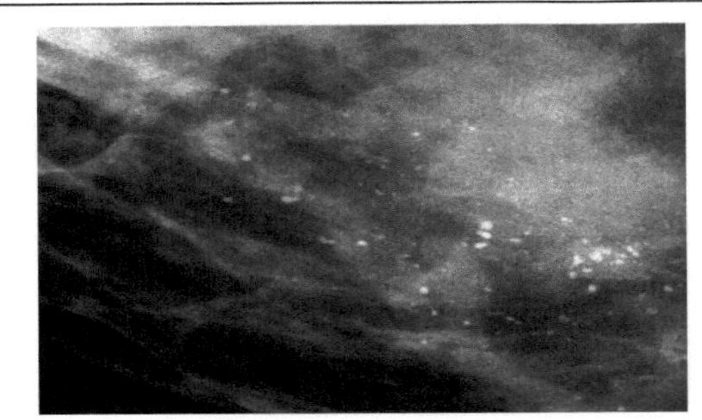

Fig. 52. Hyperplasia ductal hyperplasia hyperplasia. Mammogram. Numerous round calcifications, some of which are dusty.

2.2. Atypical Lobular Hyperplasia

Atypical lobular hyperplasia is an epithelial proliferation of ductulo-lobular units containing cellular atypia with characteristics similar to lobular cancer in situ. A lesion at risk of malignant degeneration, the relative risk of breast cancer is multiplied by 4 compared with the general population and multiplied by 8 in women with a first-degree family history.They are often discovered by chance during a histological examination. They are often asymptomatic, but can take the form of palpable masses. On mammography, imaging is non-specific and all types of microcalcifications are found, including amorphous, polymorphous, punctiform or rounded, masses and architectural deformities (fig. 53).

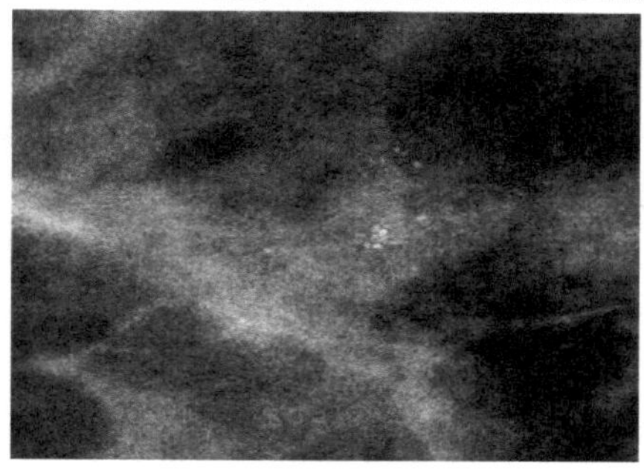

Fig. 53. atypical lobular hyperplasia. Mammogram. Focus of numerous dusty calcifications with a few polymorphic calcifications (arrow).

3.Malignant breast diseases and calcifications

3.1. Lobular carcinoma in situ (LCIS)

Lobular carcinoma in situ is characterised by a proliferation of small, loosely cohesive cells with regular, rounded nuclei in the breast lobules. Multiple or bilateral sites are common.

Lobular carcinomas in situ account for around 10-15% of breast cancers in situ. They have no specific radiological manifestation and are discovered incidentally during histological analysis of associated benign lesions. CLIS are essentially microcalcifications (in about 95% of cases) of all types, rarely a round mass or architectural disorganisation (fig. 54).

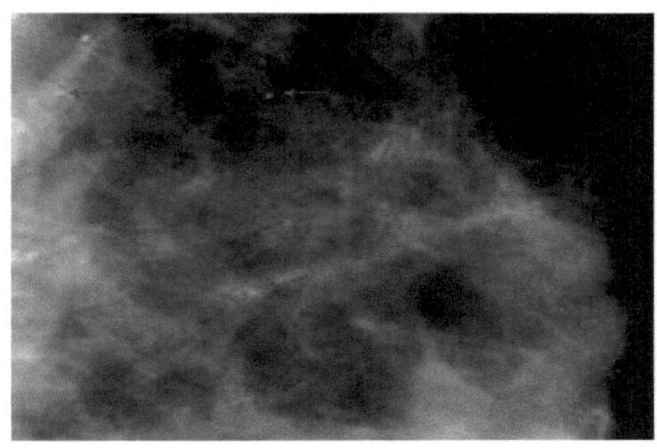

Fig. 54. Carcinoma lobular in situ. Mammography. Microcalcifications irregular, polymorphic, few numerous (arrows) [16].

3.2. Ductal carcinomas

Most carcinomas found in the presence of microcalcifications are of the galactophore type, known as intracanal carcinomas.
Ductal carcinomas are a heterogeneous group comprising lesions of varying degrees of aggressiveness.
There are two types of ductal carcinoma:

- intracanal carcinoma of the comedogenic type or comedocarcinoma;
- non-comedogenic intracanal carcinoma.

Ductal carcinomas of all types are either strictly limited to the wall of the galactophore, in which case they are known as in situ carcinomas, or they cross the basal membrane of the galactophore, in which case they are known as infiltrating carcinomas.
In general, comedogenic carcinomas generate more foci of microcalcifications than non-comedogenic carcinomas. Nevertheless, all of these carcinomas can result in foci of microcalcifications.

3.2.1. Ductal carcinoma in situ (DCIS)

Ductal carcinoma in situ accounts for 85-90% of breast cancers in situ, and thanks to the rise in screening, its rate has reached 15-20% of cancers [17]. It is a heterogeneous group, combining lesions with different cytological, architectural, biological and evolutionary aspects. The majority of ISCCs are thought to arise at the junction between the lobules and the terminal milk duct and to spread from proximal to proximal, towards the nipple, but also retrogradely, colonising the mammary lobules.Several classifications have been proposed, distinguishing three classes of ISCC with increasing aggressiveness. They are based mainly on nuclear grade and/or the presence of necrosis, but none of them has become established despite the various consensus meetings [18].In around 5 to 15% of cases, there is no mammographic abnormality, and CCIS is often discovered by chance during surgery or in the presence of a clinical abnormality (bloody uniporic nipple discharge, Paget's disease) [19].
On mammography [20-22], the most frequent sign of CCIS is a focus of microcalcifications, in 75% to 90% of cases. The microcalcifications have two origins, either secretory (well-differentiated low-grade or intermediate-grade CCIS), of unsuspicious morphology, round and powdery in 57% of cases, or

linked to tumour cell necrosis (high-grade CCIS), essentially irregular, vermicular, punctiform microcalcifications. The shape and distribution of the calcifications (non-round focus, segmental or linear distribution) are most often elements in favour of CCIS (figs. 55, 56).

Other mammographic abnormalities are much less frequent. They may include an irregularly shaped mass (< 10% of cases), architectural distortion (< 10 of cases).

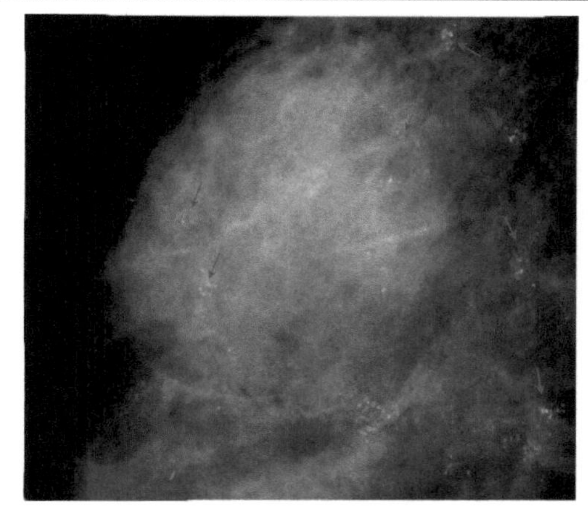

Fig. 55. Ductal carcinoma in situ. Mammogram. Multiple foci of amorphous and polymorphous microcalcifications (arrows).

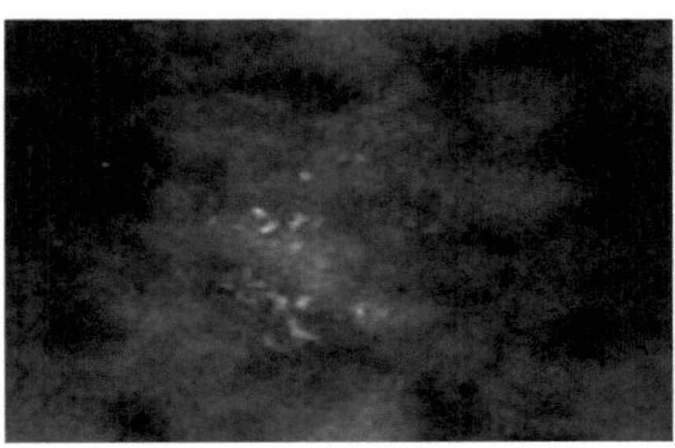

Fig. 56. Ductal comedocarcinoma in situ. Mammogram. Focal point of polymorphic microcalcifications.

3.2.2. Non-specific infiltrating carcinoma

Ductal carcinoma, or non-specific carcinoma according to the new nomenclature of the World Health Organisation [23], is a clonal proliferation of epithelial cells originating from the ductal-lobular end units, with extension of the tumour cells through the basement membrane. It accounts for 70-80% of invasive cancers.

On mammography, a mass with spiculated borders is found in around 70% of cases. It is frequently associated with microcalcifications, the characteristics of which are similar to those of CCIS. They may present as isolated foci of microcalcifications or when they extend over more than 4 cm (fig. 57, 58).

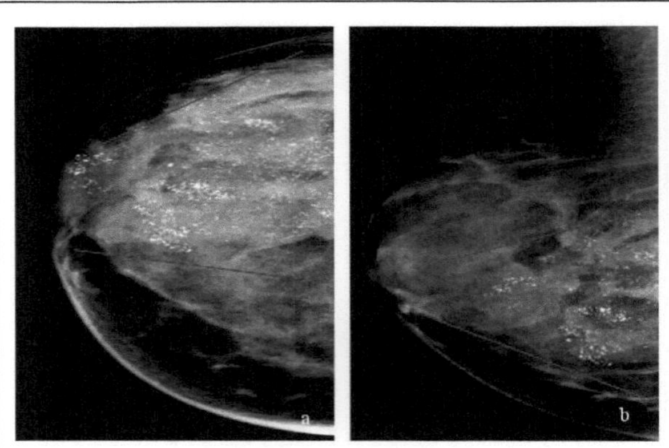

Fig. 57. Non-specific infiltrating carcinoma. Mammogram (a) frontal view (b) oblique view. Polymorphic microcalcifications with a few coarsely heterogeneous microcalcifications, arranged segmented.

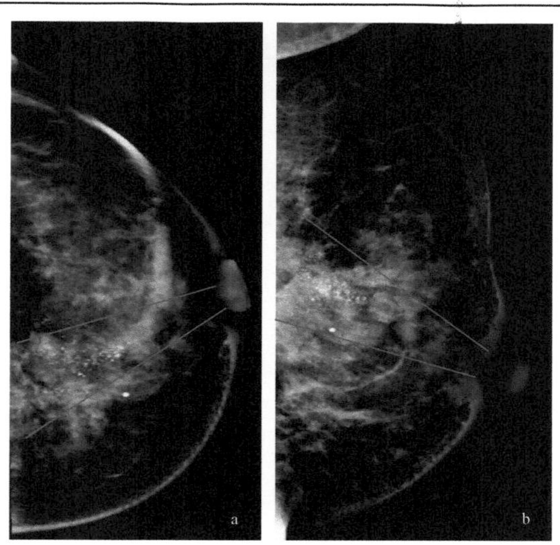

Fig. 58. Non-specific infiltrating carcinoma. Mammography (a) frontal view (b) oblique view. Polymorphic microcalcifications associated with coarse, heterogeneous microcalcifications of segmented.

3.3. Invasive lobular carcinoma

Invasive lobular carcinoma is an epithelial proliferation of the lobular type with extension of the tumour cells to the basement membrane. It accounts for less than 5 to 15% of invasive cancers. It is often asymptomatic, but may present as a palpable mass.On mammography, it usually presents as a dense spiculated mass or as architectural asymmetry. Microcalcifications are rare in this type of carcinoma and vary from 1 to 16% depending on the series [24, 25]. They are non-specific and of all types (Fig. 59).

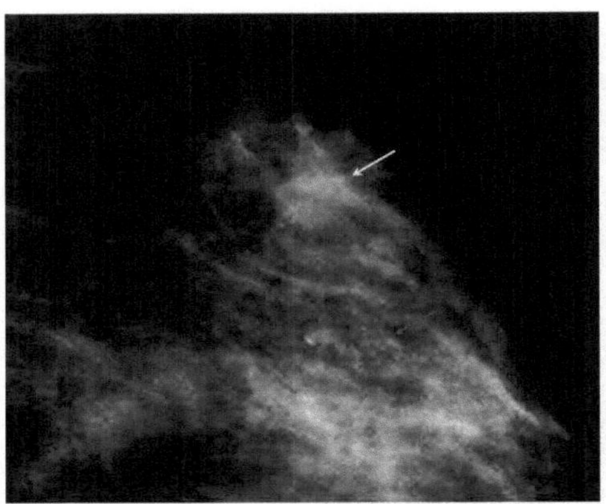

Fig. 59. Invasive lobular carcinoma. Mammogram. Spiculated mass (white arrow) associated with a few dusty microcalcifications (red arrow).

REFERENCES

1.Couturaud B, Fitoussi A. Anatomy / surgery of breast cancer. Conservative treatment, oncoplasty. Surgical techniques in gynaecology. Elsevier Masson; 2011 ; 4-7.

2.Frappart L, Boudeulle M, Boumendil J, Hu Chi L, Martinon I, Paladyer C et al. Structure and composition of microcalcifications in benign and malignant lesions of the breast. Human Pathol 1984; 15: 880-889.

3.Frappart L, Remy I, Hu Chi L, Bremond A, Raudrant D, Grousson B et al. Different types of microcalcifications observed in breast pathology. Correlations with histopathological diagnosis and radiological examination of operative specimens. Virchows Arch 1986; 410: 179-187.

4.Galkin BM, Feig SA, Patchesky AS et al. Ultrastructure and microanalysis of "benign" and "malignant" breast calcifications. Radiology 1977; 124: 245-249.

5.Baur A, Bahrs SD, Speck S, Wietek BM, Kremer B, Vogel U, et al. Breast MRI of pure ductal carcinoma in situ: sensitivity of diagnosis and influence of lesion characteristics. Eur J Radiol 2013;82:1731-7.

6.Hammersleya JA, Partridgeb SC, Blitzera GC, Deitcha S, Rahbarb H. Management of high-risk breast lesions found on mammogram or ultrasound: the value of contrast-enhanced MRI to exclude malignancy. Clinical Imaging 49; 2018; 174-180. https://doi.org/10.1016/j.clinimag.2018.03.011

7.Andolina VF, Lill√© SL, Willison KM, Mammographic Imaging. A practical guide. 2 nd ed. Lippincott Williams and Wilkins; 2001.

8.Austin C. R and Short R. V. Hormonal Control of Reproduction. 2nd edition of Reproduction in Mammals, Vol.3. Cambridge: Cambridge University Press. 1984.

9.Faulconer LS, Parham CA, Connor DM, Kuzmiak C, et al. Effect of breast compression on lesion characteristic visibility with diffraction-enhanced imaging. Acad Radiol 2010; 17 (4) : 433-40. Epub 2009 Dec 29.

10. Kinzelin S. Positioning, the √©tape cl√© of the mammography examination. Imagerie du sein Elsevier Masson, 2012; 2: 19-27.

11. Mancuso S, Ottolenghi G. The oblique projection in the radiologic Study of the breast. Minerva Ginecol 1989; 41 (7): 325-8.

12. Konguth PJ, Rimer BK, Conaway MR, et al. Impact of patient-controlled compression on the mammography experience. Radiology 1993; 186 (1): 99-102.

13. Muntz EP, Logan WW, Focal spot size. And scatter supression in magnification mammography. AJR Am J Roentgenol 1979; 133 (3): 453-9.

14. D'Orsi CJ et al. ACR BI-RADS ¬Æ Atlas, Breast Imaging Reporting and Data System. Reston, VA, American College of Radiology; 2013.

15. Frouge C,Guinnebretière JM, Contessor et al.Physiopathology of breast microcalcifications.Feuillets de radiologie1994;34: 370-8.

16. Lévy L, Michelin J, Teman G, Martin B, Lacan A, Dana A and Meyer D. Diagnosis of mammary microcalcifications. Encycl Méd Chir (Elsevier, Paris), Radiodiagnosis - Urology-Gynaecology, 34-825-A-10, 1999, 27 p.

17. Virning BA, Tuttle TM, Shamliyan T, Kane RL. Ductal carcinoma in situ of the breast: a systematic review of incidence, treatment, and outcomes. J Natl Cancer Inst 2010; 102(3): 170-8.

18. Consensus conference on the classification of ductal carcinima in Situ. Cancer 1997; 80(9): 1789-802.

19. INCa. Recommendations and guidelines: in situ breast cancer. Boulogne-Billancourt : INCa; 2009.

20. Heywang-Köbrunner SH,Schreer I, Dershaw D, Grumbach Y. Imagerie diagnostique du sein. Mammography, ultrasound, MRI, interventional techniques. Paris: Masson; 2000.

21. Travade A, Isnard A, Grimbergue H. Imagerie de la pathologie mammaire. Paris : Masson; 1995.

22. Hagay C, Chérel P, de Maulmont C, Ouhioun O, Nodiot P, Plantet MM. Management of microcalcifications. J Le Sein 2001; t.11 (1-2) : 79-99.

23. Lakhani SR, Ellis IO, Schnitt SJ, Tan PH, van de Vijver MJ (Eds.): WHO Classification of Tumours of the Breast. IARC: Lyon 2012.

24. Harvey JA. Unusual breast cancers: useful clues to expanding the differential diagnosis. Radiology 2007;242:683-94.

25. Le Treut A, Jeantet B, Boisserie-Lacroix M, Trojani M. Tubular carcinomas of the breast: radio-clinical aspects. Rev Im Med 1991;(3-4):257-60.

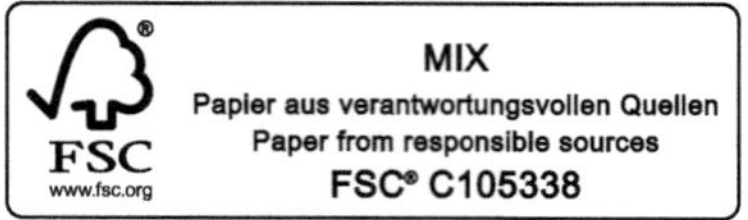

Printed by Books on Demand GmbH, Norderstedt / Germany